HOW TO LOSE 10 POUNDS IN A WEEK

The Ultimate 7 Day Weight Loss Kick-Start for Optimum Health

EMMA GREEN

Book

2

"I love everything about Emma's connection to weight loss and health."

Hi, my name is Nat Lee, and I've spent most of my life looking pretty good and feeling great. That was up until I started eating on the run and allowing my busy life as a mom to take hold of me. While working too.

In truth, I knew I should eat great food, but time constraints and "motherly craziness" got the better of me. I made sure my son ate well. But I didn't, which was silly, really. Parenting is one of those things that just takes over your life, I suppose. So, anyway, I kinda ate loads of stuff I shouldn't, and drank sodas and milkshakes an awful lot. Chocolate and takeout became my best friend, and I became overweight, by anyone's standards. No one really told me I looked bad, I mean, most people aren't that obvious. But when I was diagnosed with a severe illness and bedridden for four years, it became time to do something to help my recovery. I made the change as soon as I could.

Since reading Emma's books, I've lost 18.5 kg (which is 40 amazing pounds). And I've managed to keep it off by following her wonderful advice, and by using her awesome, easy-to-do recipes. I live relatively simply, but her guide to nutrition and her tips and tricks have helped me a bucket load. Thank you Emma, you've literally changed my life!

CONTENTS

INTRODUCTION

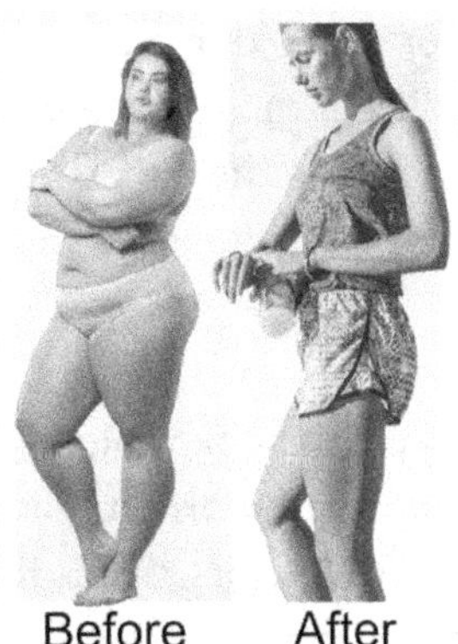

Hi! And thanks so much for joining me here. My name is Emma Green and I've lost over 100 pounds on my journey, so far! I can't wait to share my knowledge with you, so you can benefit from it, too! We can do this together.

Some of my best secrets can be found in my title, "How I Lost 100 Pounds! My Personal Weight Loss Strategies for Optimum Happiness." You can see exactly what I did over a 22-month period to lose the weight for good... and keep it off. I now feel better and happier than I've ever felt before. And I wish there was a book like it when I was at my heaviest; most-lowest point. You will learn about the purposeful nutrition, balance as a way of eating, a great ancient technique to skyrocket your weight loss, how to lose belly fat, superfoods and herbs, and all about water weight and cellulite removal and prevention. It's totally FREE! Please feel free to pick up your copy today.

Growing up, I learned to love my southern lifestyle. It was cheaper to eat badly than it was to get fresh produce at the time. We didn't have heaps of money and we got by as best we could. So, my mom got what was cheap when we ventured to the local store. The food was inexpensive, and my mother made us the best meals, despite us living below the poverty line. When you're poor, you tend to eat more calorie-dense foods because they're actually cheaper than fruits and vegetables, and that's just how it was for us. I don't blame Mom for spoiling me, because, in reality, she didn't know any better. The only difference nowadays, is that we are noticing the effects that modern day (westernized) diets have on the body as a whole.

Losing 10 pounds in one week is achievable, as long as you do the right things. We need to take the guess work out, and once we do that, then we can achieve real, definitive results. **It should also be noted that starving yourself is not going to help** (or make you feel any better) by the end of it. Healthy (purposeful) eating along the way is a more natural way to lose weight and is much better for your body in the long run, as well.

To lose 10 pounds in one week, you need to **focus on both nutritional needs and water weight.** This means that you will have to reduce your liquid intake and consume highly nutritious foods well-known in one particular diet style.

Exercise used to be known as an important factor, but it's not needed as a major player, actually. An increase in vigorous activities, sports, general movement, and aerobic exercise are not crucial – not anymore. And this is super-important. There are a few more tips and tricks too, so let's get started, shall we? It's really great to have you here. Welcome! Let's go...

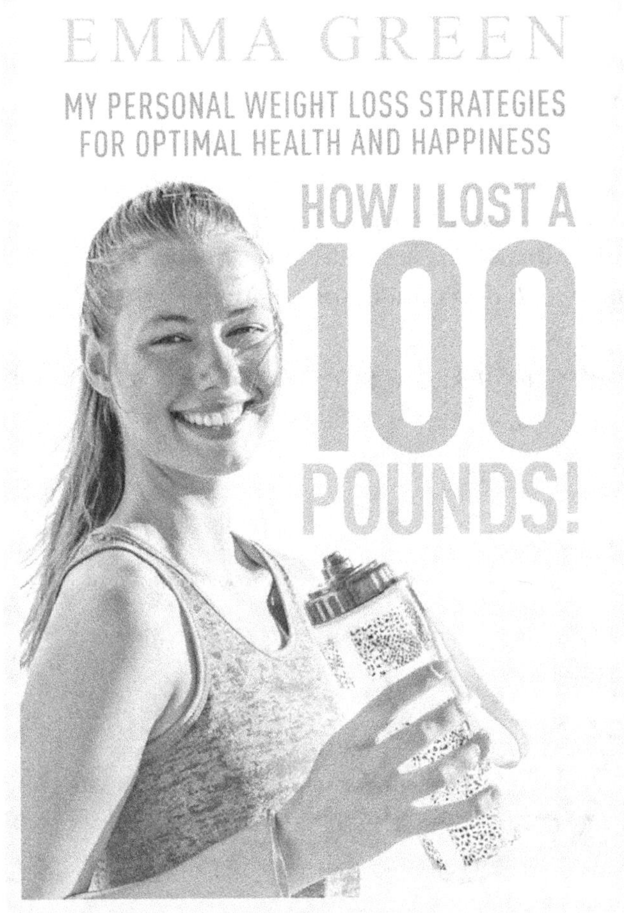

Btw check out "How i lost a 100 pounds" if you haven't already, its got loads of value and its completely FREE :)

FREE GIFTS!

Here are 3 bonus books I want to gift you for coming and reading this title! Sign up to my newsletter and you will receive:

Weight Loss Myths - 9 myths that you are mostly likely doing right now that are totally pointless and are a waste of time toward your weight loss goals.

How to Lose Weight Fast – A 10 day plan I personally put together to make that weight literally melt before your eyes (it worked for me!)

And... Weight Loss Secrets - Secrets the main stream media and health industry never talk about because (let's be honest) things that work don't make them money!

Click here to sign up! or for paperback versions grab it through the ebook completely FREE!

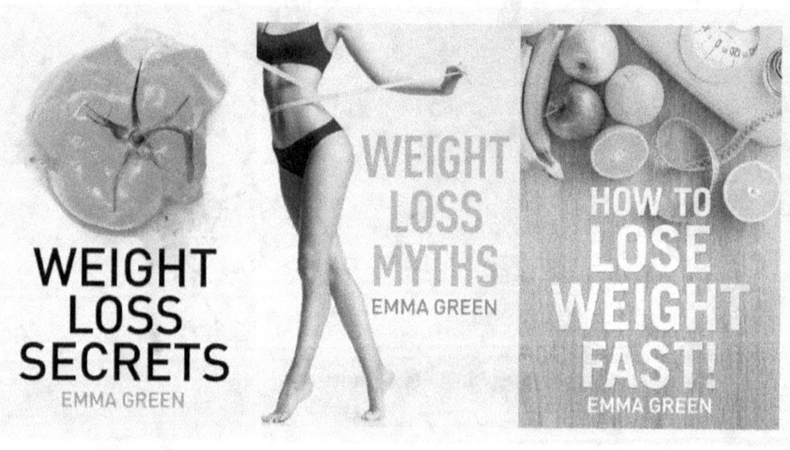

Chapter One

U.S. STATISTICS SHOW OBESITY IS RISING

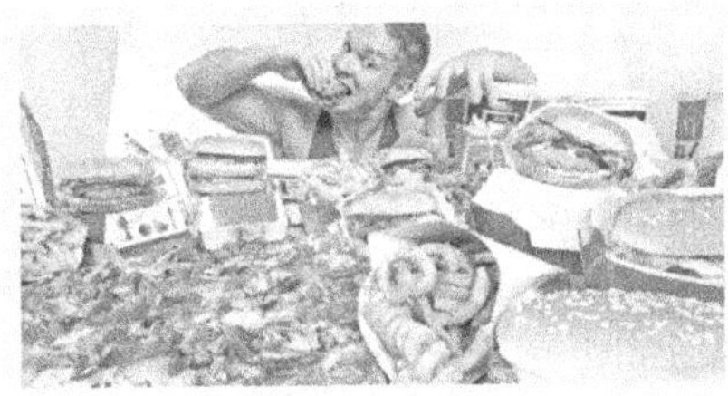

Obesity in the U.S. is a significant problem, and it is an issue that shows no signs of slowing down, unfortunately. Recent studies have (again) confirmed the trend in the number of Americans who are obese. And this number is growing each year, and has been for the past three decades.

One of the latest studies that was conducted by the Center for Disease Control and Prevention shows that almost 40% of adults in America are obese. What is even more alarming, is that the study showed a figure of nearly 20% of U.S. adolescents is also obese. These numbers are the highest figures ever recorded and appear to get worse with each survey that is conducted.

Long-term health (which is associated with these figures) is worrisome because it shows that one in five children from the age of 6-11 years is obese; as is the statistic that shows one in five children aged 12-19 years is, as well. These are staggering statistics. If this isn't bad enough, the study has also shown that one in ten preschool-aged children are also obese, not just overweight.

What is Obesity?

This is the medical term for an individual who has a body mass index of 30, or above. The findings from these latest studies in the U.S. further support reports from the World Health Organization that show childhood obesity around the world is also a growing problem, and one that has increased by tenfold over the last forty years.

When children become obese or become overweight, the chances are they will stay in this state and will be exposed to higher chances of dying earlier during adulthood.

Why Are So Many People Obese?

The Department of Agriculture made a report that showed that the average American consumed around 20% more calories per year than they did in earlier years. Much of this comes with the increase in meat consumption. Nowadays, Americans consume a figure of around 195 lbs. of meat, compared to a value of 138 lbs. during the 1950s.

With this increase in meat consumption comes an increase in added fats that are consumed, with figures rising by two thirds over the same period. This coupled with the lack of necessary exercise, means that individuals have gained weight over the period of time. In the past four decades, grain consumption in America has grown by 40% as an additional leverage factor.

One of the main contributors to the rise in obesity is fast food. This is directly related to an individual's body mass index. An average American diet consists of around 11% fast food. With this, comes lots of added sugars from soda and energy drinks which wreak havoc on a person's waistline. Not to mention the overload of calories found within each meal.

Mixed Messages for Nutrition

We can now see that it's not only the amount of food that is eaten, but also "what" is eaten that affects a person's overall health. Some mixed messages are given to Americans about what to eat - and by how much.

There is the up-sizing of meals, processed meals, and the drive-thru fast food availability that are portrayed as both delicious and cheap.

Additionally, adults now spend more time working, and less time at home in the kitchen than they used to. It is easy to see why grabbing a slice of cold pizza and having a diet drink for lunch appears to be the best route to take. It's fast and easy. Too easy.

Chapter Two

HOW TO LOSE 10 POUNDS IN 1 WEEK

When I finally discovered that I could lose weight effectively, I weighed myself on a Monday at 7 am. I wanted to know if I could lose a big number in one week. My aim was 5 pounds. Although, I was hoping for 7. I was eating well and using the keto style of dieting (and some paleo.) I was utilizing the stomach rubbing technique, bike riding for 20 minutes a day, and using juicing and smoothies as my substitute for breakfast. I watched my fluid intake and kept it to the bare minimum (6 cups for the day).

When I re-weighed myself, I had lost 11.5 pound in one week; over double what I had planned to lose. I was literally speechless. I jumped for joy like you see them doing in silly TV commercials.

Individuals who go on a standard diet can lose 1 to 2 pounds per week. Aiming to lose 10 pounds in one week seems to be out of reach, but it can be done. In this book we will go through all the the methods i used to lose that 11.5 pounds in a week.

Ultimately, we want to achieve weight loss safely, always. If you have any questions or concerns, you should always consult a professional if you need more information.

Overview

Basically, there are two distinct parts of how to plan your action that will help you to lose this amount of weight in such a short space of time. This can be broken down into **utilizing ketogenic nutrition as a major focus** and **adding the 6-cup rule** (discussed in the water weight chapter), which both go hand-in-hand and work together to allow you to reach your goal. In addition, using **light exercise, green smoothies/juicing** and using **superfoods and herbs** can also help to aid in real weight loss, and, especially to aid the body with great nutrients while it sheds this weight.

As you are aiming to lose ten pounds quickly, you will have to drastically slash the number of carbohydrates you consume on a daily basis. By doing this, you can utilize the **ketogenic style** of eating (discussed soon), so you can set your body on track with nutrition that's in complete parallel to your weight loss goal. The ketogenic style of eating **utilizes the fats for energy** burning as opposed to sugar, which are usually utilized in most westernized eating plans.

Ketogenic Nutrition

We want to create a balance of:

Low Carbohydrates – 5% (or lower) of your daily intake will be made up of carbs.

Protein – Between 15% and 35% of your daily intake will be made up of protein.

High Fat - Between **60% - 80%** of your daily intake will be made up of fat.

When you follow these ratios, real weight loss can happen. Your body is depleted of glucose, and it ramps up its production of **ketones** which are then used to **produce energy**.

The human body holds up to 500 grams of carbohydrates in the form of glycogen, and it is this glycogen that carries three times the weight of water. So, with the reduction in insulin levels from diet change, the kidneys will flush away excess sodium which leads to less water retention as a major reduction addition.

Now, with the reduction in water weight and a reduced body fat, you will lose the weight. This is because there will be less intestinal waste and food which has not been digested, along with fiber within the digestive system.

In addition, the reduced carbohydrate intake can also lead to significant amounts of weight loss from any excess water in the body, and body fat, as well. Read this entire book to learn more on diet styles and water weight reduction techniques.

Aid Water Weight

It's important to understand that while trying to lose this much weight in one week, a fair amount will come from **water weight**, and water weight is covered soon in a chapter on just that. **We need to stay at a 6-cup limit per day, for all fluids, including those found in foods.** Added with the ketogenic diet, the body's insulin levels will also drop which will force your body into shedding stored carbs which hold water, as well.

Chapter Three

WATER WEIGHT AND CELLULITE

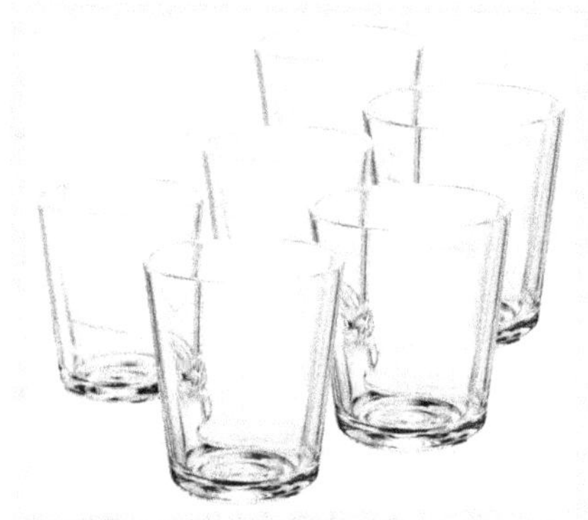

When I first read the truth about water weight... the penny dropped so well for me. I'd always thought that I was "big boned" or "had a thyroid issue," of some kind. I couldn't understand why I had a bloated look about me. And the terribly-awful cellulite that made up most of me, unfortunately.

Through college, I drank sodas, and milkshakes, and water, and tea, and coffee. It was like "liquid city" for me! It was cool to have drinks with friends too. It was part of my social life. "Wanna grab a coffee?" was the usual invitation. You know the drill. Anyway, I consumed (at that point) a gobsmacking 14 cups of liquid a day; not including the foods I consumed. This was before I made a change.

But... even when I researched weight loss, every single health book and website I looked at said, "Drink plenty of fluids to flush out the toxins," or something similar to that. And this led to an ever-increasing vicious cycle that meant I held onto water weight. And water (if it can't escape) turns into cellulite, over time. Aha! Problem finally solved...

Much emphases are placed on losing weight by what you eat and exercise, yet it is also important to look at the effects that water (and other fluids) have on the body. It is essential to remain hydrated, especially if you are consuming higher amounts of fiber. But, more importantly, there is an impact on health if you drink too much, as well. On top of that, there is the weight that fluids have and how they will affect your goal of achieving a ten-pound weight loss in one week.

Cellulite... a wonderful addition to my thighs (in the past, thank goodness). I used to joke about it with friends and wonder how they didn't have it. My best friend Elise never had a weight problem; she also never drank or ate as much as me. I could eat 6 to 7 slices of pizza and down 2 sodas all in one sitting. She couldn't believe how much I consumed. So, you'll love this section, and it helped me so much. I never really knew what I was doing to my body, and this explains a lot. I hope you get great information from practicing it.

The advice in this chapter comes from a **Taoist practice** that has been used for many thousands of years. It has stood the test of time, and it is another way you can get your body back on track and lose that ten pounds in one week, which is the goal of this title.

The kidneys in the body have the function of filtering waste water from the blood. A lot of how much water the kidneys are capable of filtering out relates to the effectiveness of your kidneys' performance for this task.

Healthy kidneys can filter (on average) 6 cups of water in any twenty-four-hour period, and if they are pushed to filter larger quantities than this, they become overworked and will weaken, over time.

If you have healthy kidneys and you consume this six cups of water (maximum) per day, you will be on a level conducive to health. However, if you drink more than this (and what your kidneys can efficiently handle), this fluid remains in the body and travels back around the bloodstream. It can only be eliminated through perspiration. Up until that time, it stays in the body and will be carried around as excess weight.

As you have set your goal on losing ten pounds in one week, and because you have to embark on a lot more exercise for the duration, perspiration will not be a problem, although, you will only be discarding the excess amounts of water. And this leads to another issue. Because you might only lose a proportion of the water levels inside your body, any incoming water or fluids will back up the levels, and they become retained in the skin. Once there is enough buildup of water, the skin bloats so it can accept this water (that is ready to be released through perspiration).

However, the remaining water can become stagnant and holds a lot of waste products and toxins. Once this waste accumulates, it can be considered as "urine," and it has the potential to remain in these areas for any period - either a day, a week, or even years.

Once there is this buildup of water in the body, it transforms into a mucus-like substance. It is still water, although it is in a thicker (more-solid) form. When individuals experience this, they think they have added fat, yet it might be this mucus that is stuck in-between the body tissues. Once this stagnant water has turned into mucus and then hardens further, it turns into what we know as cellulite.

Cellulite; and Getting Rid of It

Because this cellulite is not really water and it is not really body fat either, the question is, how do we get rid of it? Perspiration from exercise is not a means of removing cellulite on its own. Only fresh water can be released through perspiration.

There are two ways that cellulite can be reduced and removed, the first and **simplest way is to reduce your fluid intake (drink less) to six cups**, or less, per day. For the whole process, this is the most critical part.

The second step is to stimulate these cellulite deposits and break them up. Two of the most comfortable ways of doing this is by having a hot bath or by taking a sauna.

The best way to get rid of these deposits is to heat them up and break them down. In simple terms, the more they are massaged, the more they will break up and can then be eliminated. Once you do this (while the body is hot), the pores will open and allow for a much more significant amount of perspiration.

The 6-Cup (Per Day) Rule

When people are trying to lose weight by whatever means, there is a good chance they cut out the junk foods. They might even have a salad for dinner, accompanied by a glass of water, as an example.

This can lead to a miscalculation of water intake as salad contains water which has to be purified by the kidneys. When 6 cups of water (liquid) per day is the maximum, this includes anything that might hold water.

Fruits, vegetables, soups, and any beverages all go toward this total. It is a little hard to calculate when you consume foods which contain water, and this is another area where juicing and green smoothies can come to the rescue. Essentially, because you can measure these - so the liquids in the fruits and vegetables can be accounted for.

Chinese medicine leads us to know that kidney problems are highlighted by symptoms such as gout. This is a buildup of uric acid which crystallizes in the joints where inflammation occurs.

Water Retention and Kidney Problems

For you to have an indication of if your kidneys are performing at their most efficient capacity, you can follow these guidelines that will highlight if you might have water retention - and that your kidneys are not working efficiently.

If you have cellulite, this is the most straightforward sign to show your kidneys are not able to perform as they should. If you are retaining water, you can check areas which most commonly form cellulite, and these are the buttocks, belly, thighs, and the upper arms where you get flabby tissues that sit underneath the skin.

Rapid weight changes are also an indication. This would be losing or gaining as much as 5 lbs. in a day, or two. If this occurs, this has to be water retention (or severe water loss) because fat is unable to form that quickly.

You can press your finger into the skin of your arm or your leg. When you remove it and there is a white mark on your skin for a second or two, this indicates water retention. If your body has little or no water retention, the mark vanishes immediately, or there is no mark showing at all. The more extended the period the mark remains, the more water retention your body has.

Physicians and Water Retention

If you think you have water retention and you visit a physician, their first usual cure for this is the use of diuretic tablets. These can get rid of water, yet there is one problem with this way of working. Your kidneys are not performing as they should, so putting more strain on them to flush more fluids from the body will only make things worse.

The doctor might also advise drinking plenty of water to flush out the system. This leads to a situation where you have two, "problem solutions" to get rid of fluids, yet you are drinking more fluids than your body can eliminate.

It is much healthier to limit your fluids to 6 cups a day, and then either take hot baths or a sauna and break down the cellulite once and for all, by utilizing the use of massage. All this can be done with no wear and tear on your kidneys.

Being aware of the fluids you consume and how they can adversely affect your body is crucial. If you do it correctly, this is an excellent means of losing weight as an accompaniment to the keto way of eating.

If you exercise a lot and you perspire, you should not be tempted to go over your 6-cup limit unless you absolutely need to, always follow the signals of the body. Although it might appear what you are doing is the right thing to do, you are not going to get rid of this excess water and hit your goal of ten pounds in one week.

Water can be a dieter's best friend, yet it can also stop your diet from even working - without you knowing it. So, count all fluids for the 6-cup rule. Your kidneys will thank you!

Chapter Four

THE MYTH OF COUNTING CALORIES

Burn more Calories Than You Consume – This is Impossible!

Regardless of what method or diet you followed in the past, this **used to be known** as the true secret of weight loss. You were told, "There is no way around it," and although the theory sounds simple, it doesn't actually work well at all.

In truth, I did this so much! It drove me crazy counting every piece of food and every drink! I thought I was made up of numbers. Like a strange math puzzle or something. When I realized through my research efforts that balance was key... I stopped doing it! I literally couldn't cope with the numbers game anymore, and my friend Elise said, "Oh, thank God, I was going to slap you soon!" Of course, she was only joking, but I was so thankful when I focused more on portion size. It was so much easier and made me feel freer in my plan.

One pound is equal to 3,500 calories, so losing ten pounds in one week means that you'd need to burn about 5000 calories per day for the 7-week period!!! This figure lessens to **4200 for women and men, per day,** due to the decrease in calorie intake per day, of around 800 calories for each gender. **But, the recommended new calorie intake would be 1200 calories per day, for women, and 1700 calories per day, for men,** approximately. Imagine trying to eat that little... and do over 4 hours of exercise per day?? **It's just not a workable option,** and it doesn't work anyway, because the body becomes fatigued and usually places fat around the middle section of the body to compensate. It's also not good to stress the heart by crazily exercising, either.

You were probably told, "The calories will be burned from any activity you do" - and not just purposeful exercise. Breathing, walking around, or even climbing stairs are all going to contribute toward this magical number value of 4,200 calories!! **It's craziness to think of even doing this to your body.** It is a massive contribution, but it is a contribution, nonetheless. No way, it's not okay!! We don't need to do it.

You Were Probably Told, "Knowing the Goal is a Challenge"

Even before you started a ridiculous calorie counting/exercise game, you already know it is going to be difficult, because burning the necessary calories in a day this way, **would be** a lot of hard work. **Crazy-hard!!** A prime example is a person who weighs 160 lbs. They would burn around 1,000 calories playing a highly competitive sport for 90 minutes. If you calculate this, **you would have to play this sport for six plus hours to burn the 4,200 calories. #OMG!!! No!**

The Old Theory Was Based on What an Average Person Consumes in Calories

An average woman will usually consume around 2,000 calories per day, and the average man will consume 2,500 calories, approximately. So, if you continue with this figure, you will neither lose weight, or gain weight (was the old thought on this). So, we were told that when you are aiming to lose weight, and you reduce your calorie intake to around 1,200 calories (women) and 1700 (men) per day, a difference of 800 calories is given. And so now you need to only burn **4,200 (women and men)**. We already worked out that six hours of vigorous exercise would need to be maintained daily!!! **This is impossible unless you are an athlete training for The Olympic Games?**

Other Weight Loss Myths

Before moving to the diet section, there are a few myths you might have heard, and these described are most-definitely false.

Myth #1 Any Calorie Is the Same

A calorie is a unit of energy, and that much is true. However, how these calories or units of energy affect your body is very different. Varying foods pass through various metabolic pathways and affect hormones that regulate body weight and hunger.

A good example is consuming 100 calories of chocolate. This would have a much more significant and negative impact on your body than 100 calories worth of healthy salad. Additionally, a protein calorie is not the same as a carb or a fat calorie. The body utilizes the vitamins and minerals in certain foods differently. So, we need to stay with foods that boost vitality, and aid in weight loss, not fat storage, as a necessity.

Myth #2 You Will Lose Weight Every Day

This is not true, some days you will go up a little, and other days you will drop to compensate. This is one reason they say not to weigh yourself every day. In the case of women, they might have more water retention during their menstrual cycle.

Myth #3 Supplements Help to Lose Weight

Most supplements, when studied against their claims of weight loss, are shown as not as effective as their claims make out. Most people fall for marketing, and they fall under a placebo effect where they are conscious of what they eat as a result. It's usually not due to the product being viable, though.

Myth #4 Carbs Will Make You Fat

It is a fact that low-carb diets will help you to lose weight, and can do so - without a dramatic reduction in calories. As long as you keep carb intake low and protein consumption high, you can lose weight, but it will take time. Not all carbs are equal. It is true that refined carbs like sugars and grains are linked to obesity, yet whole-wheat carbs are, infact, healthy.

Myth #5 Skipping Breakfast Helps Lose Weight

People who skip breakfast have been shown to weigh more than people who eat breakfast; your body needs morning fuel for a healthier lifestyle and for safe weight loss.

Myth #6 Foods Labeled "Diet" Help Lose Weight

Many types of junk food are portrayed and marketed as being healthy. These include gluten-free foods that are processed, fat-free foods, and low-fat foods. They appear healthy from the labeling, yet the actual ingredients tell a very different story.

When you count your calories, and you have reduced them, don't be tempted to cut them even further, because you will feel hungry, and you might become very irritable. That doesn't help the cause at all. The one advantage of the keto diet as part of your goal-reaching, is to make sure you feel satisfied, and that you are able to resist the urge to quit.

Chapter Five

THE EXERCISES YOU "USED TO" HAVE TO DO

No More Interval Training

To understand what interval training consists of, it is where you perform an activity with **high intensity for a short period**, and then you reduce the intensity for the remainder of the time.

A prime example of interval training is if you were running around a track. For the first lap you would run as fast as you can, and then the remaining three laps you would reduce this to a light-speed jog.

If you are not running around a track, you can follow the jog for three minutes and then push yourself for the next minute. This can be repeated to take you to a period of thirty minutes, which is the recommended minimum exercise period per day.

Say Goodbye to Cardio Machines and Other Contraptions:

See You Later Treadmills – These are used to keep your heart rate up. A pace that is fast enough and pushes you to keep you sweating.

Bye-Bye Elliptical Trainer – These simulate the effects of skiing and give the whole body a workout. They are slightly behind a treadmill in the burning calorie stakes.

No More Stationary Bike – These are like cardio machines because you can push yourself and keep those calories tumbling. The harder you push yourself, the harder the resistance.

No Need for Cross-Training

This is where several modes of exercise are used to develop a certain level of fitness. The types of training would vary between gyms, yet they have many benefits.

One Exercise You Can Do to Help the Cause

Bike riding for pleasure is great to help burn fat and boost metabolism. It works the entire body at the same time, and can be added to help shift the pounds. But, you don't need to do it for hours on end. 15 to 20 minutes a day is awesome!

FOCUS ON KETO AND WATER WEIGHT

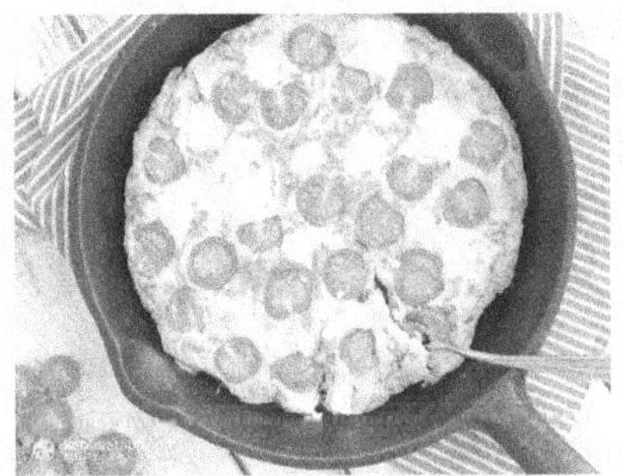

When you focus upon the ketogenic diet and the water weight (6-cup) rule, **you don't need to exercise like a machine, AT ALL.** I mean, I'm not saying you should be a couch potato, but let's take a look at what you would have to do to burn that magical number of 4200 calories!! **In the past...**

Here is an average of calories that can be burned for an individual, based on 160 lbs. in weight, as an example. All of these exercises are based on one-hour timeframes, and you **could have** mixed and matched and used them as part of your cross-training exercises for the week!! **But you won't need to!** These activities are also based on moderate performance levels, rather than vigorous or light training schedules.

Calories Burned Per Exercise Type: OUCH!!

* Outdoor Cycling – 600
* Static Cycling Gym – 700
* Stair Machine Gym – 1000
* Rowing Machine Gym – 820
* Elliptical Trainer Gym – 700
* Aerobics – 500
* Running – 800
* Jogging - 700
* Running up Stairs - 1200
* Badminton – 320
* Basketball – 450
* Boxing Punch Bag – 450
* Soccer – 680
* Martial Arts – 800
* Jump Rope – 800
* Squash – 920
* Beach Volleyball – 620
* Kayaking – 380
* Swimming, Freestyle – 550
* Swimming, Butterfly – 850
* Swimming, Leisurely – 450
* General Housework – 250
* Mowing the lawn – 450
* Raking the Lawn – 330
* Gardening – 300
* Walking – 300
* Zumba – 600

OMG! Aren't we glad we don't have to do 6 hours of those per day? Phew, me too!

Chapter Seven

THE DIET AND WHAT IT CONSISTS OF

This chapter can be broken down into sections to help divulge the information. Rather than saying eat this and don't eat that, it is to show why certain things should be eaten and others should be avoided. Knowledge is powerful.

Drinks

Water is the best thing you can drink for numerous reasons when on a diet. If you drink a large glass of water before or during a meal it will make you think you are fuller than you are, and so, you will naturally eat less and consume fewer calories.

Water also helps to keep the body hydrated and flushes out wastes and toxins from the system. There is weight in water, yet the impact on your body is far more beneficial than replacing it with drinks of other forms, apart from juicing or green smoothies.

Green tea (which is unsweetened) can be consumed on occasion, and can give you that all-important break from drinking plain water. It can also flood the body with many antioxidants that will help inside your body.

If you opt for a so-called "healthy" sports drink, these can contain up to 400 calories which make up a significant portion of your daily calorie intake.

Simple Carbohydrates

These types of carbs are the ones that cause the most problems with weight gain and should be avoided as much as possible. These are also called **refined carbs** and do not contain many nutrients for the body.

Refined carbs also get absorbed by the body more quickly, and that's because they have a high GI (glycemic index). Actually, if you've eaten any of the following, you might have experienced a rush of energy, and then you feel sluggish and lethargic later on.

- Candies, cookies, and cakes
- White bread and regular pasta
- Packaged cereals (unless made with whole grains)

Complex Carbohydrates

This type of carb is suitable to include in any form of diet or weight-loss program. These are what come from whole foods (whole wheat) and give the benefits of not only having many more nutrients, but also being beneficial because they release energy slower (low GI). Therefore, they make you feel fuller for longer. They also contain more fiber which helps in the digestive system to rid the body of wastes.

- Whole-grain bread, whole-grain pasta, and red rice

- Beans and legumes, lentils, carrots, and sweet potatoes
- Vegetables and most fruits

Some fruits are high in natural sugars

Proteins, Healthy Fats, and Low-Carbohydrate Vegetables

Every meal you eat should have a portion of protein, a low-carb source, and a fat (healthy fat) source. When you do this, you will automatically reduce the number of carbohydrates you consume.

Protein is not only good for the body because of its many nutrients and vitamins, but it has also been shown to increase the metabolism by up to 100 calories per day. Protein also has the advantage of taking away the desire for mid-meal or late-night snacking by as much as fifty percent, and you might find you automatically reduce your calorie intake by around 400 calories per day, just by adding it in. Although, calorie counting isn't a major player here.

High Protein Foods Include:

- Meat – Lean bacon, beef, pork, lamb, and chicken (no skin)
- Seafood and Fish – Trout, salmon, shrimps, prawns, and lobsters
- Eggs – Free range and omega-3 enriched
- Tofu and edamame

Low-Carbohydrate Vegetables:

- Broccoli, cauliflower, kale, spinach, cabbage
- lettuce, cucumber, celery, swiss chard

Healthy Fats:

- Avocado oil, coconut oil, and extra virgin olive oil

Breakfast, Lunches, and Dinners

You should consume three meals per day and you can include healthy snacks as long as your calorie intake is still within limits.

Some foods you can snack on which are healthy and will not affect your overall calorie intake too much are as follows:

- Rice cakes
- Fresh berries
- Greek yogurt
- Unsalted nuts
- Almond milk

No Need for a Calorie Journal

It used to be, that you were to keep a calorie journal, so you could easily keep track of your daily intake, and so you would instantly see if you are in danger of exceeding your daily limit. 1200 women, per day; and 1700 men, per day, for this one-week period. **Not anymore!!**

Fast Food Beware

This is one area of food you should avoid altogether. Fast foods are cooked in trans-fats which are "bad" for you, and they all contain high amounts of added salts and sugars.

Fast foods provide minimal nutrients, and you will find that you are hungry again later, mostly because they are offering empty carbs into your system.

When You Slip

Try to give yourself rewards that are non-food elements. Listen to music, or do a favorite hobby. The secret though, is not to go overboard and get carried away with what you are eating. It is okay to slip, but falling is different. You might also find you become more determined to succeed in your weight loss goal.

Chapter Eight

THE MAGICAL KETO CONNECTION - DO THIS!

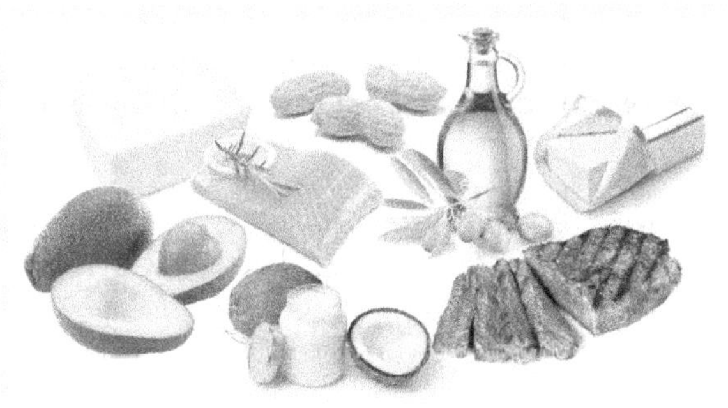

As you are aiming to lose ten pounds in one week, you will have to drastically slash the number of carbohydrates you consume on a daily basis. By doing this, you have nearly started the ketogenic diet, which is, in fact, a good thing - this diet is one of the best for losing weight quickly.

What is Keto?

The keto diet is a way of eating which promotes ketosis in the body, and to do this correctly, you follow the following ratios in your meals for the day:

Low Carbohydrates – **5% (or lower)** of your daily calories will be made up of carbs.

Moderate Protein – **Between 15% and 35%** of your daily calories will be made up of protein.

High Fat - Between **60% - 80%** of your daily calories will be made up of fat.

When you follow these ratios, something magical happens. Your body is depleted of glucose, and it ramps up its production of **ketones** which are then used to **produce energy**.

Ketosis - What Is It?

This is where the energy for the body comes from the ketones that are produced, compared to the glucose (sugar) which usually provides the energy.

It is the westernized, modern diet that provides us with high carb foods and leaves our bodies in a state of glycolysis which is bad for us. The ketogenic diet negates this, altogether.

What Are Ketones?

Ketones are the source of energy your body will use when in ketosis. These are produced by the liver when glycogen levels are very low. These ketones are a fuel supply which burns lower inside the body.

Keto and Insulin

This is the magical part of the keto connection. When you are on a high carb intake, your body produces high amounts of insulin which help carry the glucose around the body. In this state, fat deposits stay as fatty deposits and - build up over time.

When you are in ketosis, your body breaks down these fat deposits in the liver to convert to ketones, which are then used as the body's primary energy source. Not only does this help you to lose weight faster, but your insulin levels remain at a stable level rather than peaking and dropping throughout the day. This then makes it much harder for your body to store any extra fat.

Ketogenic Dietary Benefits

Weight Loss – This is the number one reason people follow a full keto diet. The body changes into a fat-burning machine.

Increased Energy Levels – The body prefers to use ketones as an energy source. You have more energy throughout the day rather than peaks and troughs.

Lessened Hunger Pangs– You will find you are less hungry when you follow this eating plan.

Cholesterol– Contrary to what was said in the past, the keto connection will lower cholesterol levels.

Diabetes and Blood Sugar – the keto diet type has been shown to have a positive effect on diabetics and blood sugar levels, overall.

WONDERFULLY-WARMING WINTER PORRIDGE: RECIPE 1

"Perfect in cooler months!"

Ingredients

- 2 tablespoons of hemp seeds
- 1/4 of a cup of walnuts or pecans, chopped
- 1/4 of a cup of coconut, flaked
- 2 tablespoon of chia seeds
- 3/4 of a cup of almond milk, unsweetened
- 1/4 of a cup of coconut milk
- 1 tablespoon of sweetener (of choice) to taste (optional)
- 1/4 of a cup of almond butter, roasted
- 1 tablespoon of coconut oil
- ½ a teaspoon of ground turmeric
- 1 teaspoon of honey
- a good pinch of ground black pepper

Instructions

- Place a skillet over medium heat.
- Add the chopped walnuts/pecans, hemp seeds and the flaked coconut.
- Roast for 1 to 2 minutes and shake or toss to prevent burning. When cooked, place in a small bowl and set aside.
- In a small saucepan, heat the almond milk and coconut milk. As it comes to a low boil, remove from the heat, carefully. Add the coconut oil, turmeric powder, black pepper, almond butter, chia seeds, and the sweetener (to taste, optional).
- Stir until well combined and set aside. Stand for 5-10 minutes. Add half of the dry roasted mix from the bowl.
- Divide the porridge into two serving bowls. Top with the remaining dry roast mix.
- Drizzle with honey or cinnamon.

KETO CRÈME FRUITY: RECIPE 2

"Extremely yummy, and easy too!"

Ingredients

- 1 tub of natural Greek yogurt
- 2 tablespoons of toasted almond flakes
- 2 tablespoons of toasted coconut flakes
- 6 tablespoons of fruit jelly, any flavor of choice can be used

Instructions

- Spoon 3 tablespoons of the fruit jelly into each serving bowl.
- Add half of the Greek yogurt into each serving bowl.
- Top with coconut flakes and almond flakes.

SPICED KETO PUMPKIN WAFFLES: RECIPE 3

"Spice and pumpkin, need I say more?"

Ingredients

- 2 eggs
- 2 tablespoons of butter, unsalted
- 2 tablespoons of heavy cream
- 1/2 a teaspoon of cinnamon powder
- 1/4 of a cup of pumpkin purée
- 1 scoop of whey protein powder, plain or vanilla
- 1 and a 1/2 tablespoons of coconut flour or almond flour
- 1 teaspoon of spiced pumpkin pie mix
- 1/4 of a teaspoon of baking soda
- 2 tablespoons of powdered sweetener (optional)
- 3 or 4 drops of vanilla extract

Instructions

- In a mixing bowl, add the eggs and whisk them together with the coconut oil, powdered sweetener (optional), and vanilla extract.

- Add the pureed pumpkin and heavy cream then whisk until you have a smooth batter.
- Add all the dry ingredients and beat together until well combined.
- Preheat waffle maker and cook mixture according to the waffle iron instructions.

ALL-DAY KETO BREAKFAST: RECIPE 4

"Awesomely-yummy and easy to do!"

Ingredients

- 2 eggs
- 6 bacon slices
- 1/2 a cup of mushrooms, fresh
- 1 avocado, peeled, pitted and sliced
- 1 tablespoon of butter, unsalted
- salt and black pepper, to taste

Instructions

- Place a skillet over medium heat, add half of butter, and then place the mushrooms top side down.
- Season with salt and pepper and cook for around 8 minutes.
- While the mushrooms are cooking, add butter to another small pan to fry the bacon and eggs to your desired liking.
- Transfer to serving plates along with the avocado slices as a garnish.

THE IMPORTANCE OF JUICING AND SMOOTHIES

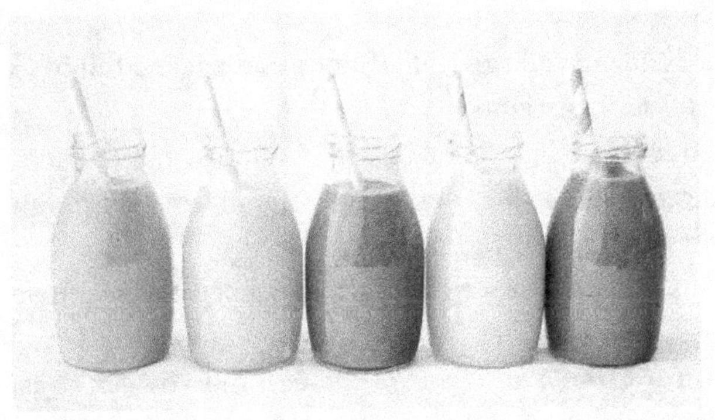

When people are aiming to lose a high amount of weight in such a short time, and they look toward keto to help them, they can become overwhelmed with the number of low-carb veggies they are required to consume. In one sitting, this can amount to a lot and for some people this can be a little too much.

One way to make sure you get more than enough vitamins, nutrients, minerals, and antioxidants into your body - is through green smoothies and juicing. These are a great way to supercharge your body, and they do nothing but help you to lose weight, while giving you maximum nutrition.

Some Great Additions to Juicing and Green Smoothies:

- **Quinoa** – Super-high in protein and fiber, as well as a host of other nutrients.
- **Cinnamon** – Full of antioxidants with anti-inflammatory properties.
- **Oats** – Low in calories and help to reduce blood pressure and are filling.
- **Chia Seeds** – High-quality protein, full of fiber and loaded with antioxidants and nutrients.
- **Spinach** – Full of vitamins and nutrients, and low in cholesterol.
- **Kale** – Low in calories, full of fiber, and packed full of vitamins and nutrients.
- **Blueberries** – Full of flavonoids, vitamins, and nutrients.
- **Bananas** – Great for energy and help improve digestion. Full of potassium and B vitamins.
- **Apples** – Great for weight loss and packed-full of nutrients to help detoxify the liver. They help with ketone production.
- **Coconut Oil** – This is one of the best oils you can consume as part of your weight loss program. It is full of healthy fats and can help to speed up your metabolism.
- **Avocado** – Packed-full of healthy nutrients; they make you feel fuller for more extended periods. Additionally, they help your body to absorb more nutrients from the other foods you eat, too.

Rotating Your Greens

When juicing and drinking green smoothies, you should make sure you rotate the greens rather than sticking with one or two of the same. This makes sure you have a broad range of health benefits in terms of the nutrient and vitamin intake.

You should take it easy on any fruits you add, as these can contain lots of natural sugars which can throw your body out of ketosis and spike your insulin levels.

Reasons Juicing and Green Smoothies are Good for You

Juicing/green smoothies are easy on the stomach and the digestion system. All the hard parts are broken down into a state that makes it easier for the body to digest, and the nutrients can work (almost immediately) without having to be broken down by the body.

Juicing/green smoothies are super-nutritious and complement the keto diet, perfectly. A good ration is to have a balance of nutrients, vitamins, and flavor where 50% are fruits and 50% green vegetables.

Two to three glasses (per day) of juicing/green smoothies is more than enough to bombard your body with nutrients and vitamins. The greener the vegetables included, the more benefits you can receive, because it is these green leaves that are packed-full of chlorophyll.

When you drink juices/green smoothies as part of your diet plan, and you follow the keto connection, you vastly reduce added salts and fats that you find in prepacked or fast foods. Everything is good and wholesome.

If you consumed vegetables which contain starch along with fruits, there might be a sensation of bloating. Juicing/green smoothies balance out the sugars which are in the fruit proportion of the smoothie.

Green Smoothies and Superfoods

While juicing and green smoothies are super-nutritious, they can be bumped up to make them a real powerhouse in the nutrient and vitamin department, and to do this, all you have to do is include some of nature's best superfoods.

These superfoods can have a dramatic effect on your weight loss, energy levels, and your overall wellbeing. You will quickly realize what you have been missing out on - just from the added energy boost.

Green Smoothie Taste

A high number of people see a green smoothie and think the taste will be horrible. If it was green leafy vegetables on their own, it might not taste the best, yet the inclusion of fruit masks the leafy flavor and makes it easier to ingest. Most are super-yummy!

How Do I Fit Juicing and Smoothies into My Plan?

As these juices/smoothies are quick and easy to make, they are ideal to use - along with a keto-styled eating plan. They are filling enough to aid one or two meals within the day, depending upon your plan.

Depending on work schedules, a useful guide is to have a super-nutritious juice/smoothie for breakfast, followed by a healthy lunch and a smoothie for dinner (or part of). Depending on your day, this can leave you space to enjoy a couple of healthy snacks, as well. This way of eating can leave you feeling satisfied, while at the same time, dropping those pounds from the number of calories you are burning.

PUNCHING-BERRY SWISS: RECIPE 1

"This is one of my all-time faves. It's great in warmer weather and you can enjoy it on ice!"

Ingredient List:

1 1/2 oz. of Swiss chard

1 persimmon - topped

5 oz. of cantaloupe

1 tablespoon of hemp seeds

1 cup of berries (amla or seasonal)

1 cup water

1 cup of ice

Directions:

When ready, simply process all the ingredients together in your favorite blender. You can shake it up or stir it up, then serve and enjoy. Cube or chop vegetables to make them blitz easier before blending. I like to add any leafy vegetables in last, and then add a touch more water if I want the consistency smoother or silkier. Great garnishes include: lemon, celery, chia seeds, or a slice of tomato. Add ice on a hot day to make the drink cooler.

LUXURY LUCUMA: RECIPE 2

"Packed with chia and spinach, you can't go wrong!"

Ingredient List:

1 1/2 oz. of baby spinach

1 orange - peeled

1 pear - chopped

1 teaspoon of lucuma

1 tablespoon of chia seeds

1 cup of water

1 cup of ice

Directions:

When ready, simply process all the ingredients together in your favorite blender. You can shake it up or stir it up, then serve and enjoy. Cube or chop vegetables to make them blitz easier before blending. I like to add any leafy vegetables in last, and then add a touch more water if I want the consistency smoother or silkier. Great garnishes include: lemon, celery, chia seeds, or a slice of tomato. Add ice on a hot day to make the drink cooler.

APPLE PECAN PARADISE: RECIPE 3

"Apples and pecans... and banana. I can't get enough of this one!"

Ingredient List:

1 1/2 oz. of baby spinach

1 banana - peeled

1 container of cinnamon applesauce - (1/2 cup)

1 tablespoon of oats

3 tablespoons of pecans

1 cup of water

1 cup of ice

Directions:

When ready, simply process all the ingredients together in your favorite blender. You can shake it up or stir it up, then serve and enjoy. Cube or chop vegetables to make them blitz easier before blending. I like to add any leafy vegetables in last, and then add a touch more water if I want the consistency smoother or silkier. Great garnishes include: lemon, celery, chia seeds, or a slice of tomato. Add ice on a hot day to make the drink cooler.

THREE GREAT JUICING RECIPES FOR YOU

GOLDEN DELICIOUS SHERBET: RECIPE 1

"Apples are always great in juices. The lemon gives it an extra tang!"

Ingredient List:

- 2 Golden Delicious apples
- 1/3 of a lemon – where possible, wax free and with the rind on

Directions:

Juice the apples and lemon, and pour over ice. Drink and enjoy adding your favorite garnish.

EFFERVESCENT TASTY: RECIPE 2

"Packed full of nutrient-rich foods. A great energy booster!"

Ingredient List:

- 3 apples
- 1 stick of celery
- half a cucumber
- spinach (1 handful)
- lettuce (1 handful)
- 2 carrots
- ice cubes

Directions:

Peel the apples and the cucumber. Dice them into cubes. Add lettuce and spinach. Add ice and blend it for a minute or so. Drink nice and cold.

LIME AND TANGO: RECIPE 3

"Pineapple makes it yummy! I really love this one!"

Ingredient List:

- 1/3 of a pineapple
- half a cucumber
- spinach (1 handful)

- 2 apples
- the juice of 2 limes
- ice cubes
- a pinch of Himalayan salt

Directions:

Juice the lime separately in juicer and pour over ice. This helps prevent oxidization of the juice. Chop pineapple and apples and add to the lime ice. Drink and enjoy.

Chapter Ten

WHY QUINOA?

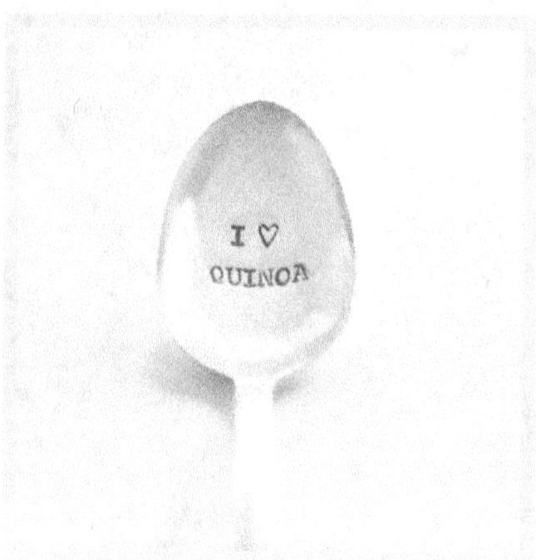

A high number of people have been on a quest to find the world's healthiest foods, and that is why we have "superfoods." There is one food that has stood out repeatedly, and this happens to be quinoa - for many reasons.

Quinoa is not a grain of any type, and it is, in fact, **a seed**, so it contains no gluten. Such is the impact quinoa has had on the world, the United Nations has stated **it is a possible food to eradicate malnutrition and hunger**. One food can do this because it contains such a broad spectrum of nutrients, and for supply, it is easy and cheap to cultivate.

What Is Quinoa?

Although the quinoa plant grows seeds rather than grains, they can be used in many of the same ways, and they are edible without much preparation. With the emergence of healthy lifestyles (the keto diet, being one), it was inevitable that quinoa would be included, and it is easy to see why. A seed that contains no gluten, yet is **power-packed with protein** and many other nutritional benefits.

Quinoa Nutrition Benefits

Quinoa is what is called a "complete protein source" which is rare, no matter what foods you eat. To simplify this, quinoa contains all 20 amino acids which include the ten essential amino acids (which the body is unable to produce on its own).

Beef that is reared on grass might contain more protein, yet as a plant-based food (and with a lot less preparation) it is ideal to include in your healthy eating plan.

When you look at the benefits that quinoa brings, you can understand why it is the one food that should not be missed from your keto-styled eating plan.

Aids in Weight Loss – Because quinoa contains a high amount of insoluble fiber and protein, it gives that full (satiated) feeling after a meal, compared to refined grains. It also spreads energy for more extended periods, so you are less likely to peak and then crash, due to insulin levels fluctuating.

A second reason it can aid in losing weight is because it contains half of your daily recommended manganese levels. These stimulate hormones and digestive enzymes. This makes it easier for the body to digest the other foods you eat.

Gluten Free – This can help many people who need to eliminate traditional grains out of their diets. Quinoa can be an excellent substitute in a good many recipes, and as an aside, it is much healthier than other forms.

These are only a couple of benefits which are directed toward anyone who is on a weight loss regime. Other benefits help in the fight against cancers, people with diabetes, and individuals who have cardiovascular illnesses. The list goes on, and you can see why it has gained so much attention over the past couple of years.

Another advantage of quinoa is its versatility, you can have it in your juicing regime, green smoothies, in salads, you can bake with it, and make health bars or cookies. There is hardly a recipe where you are not able to slip in some quinoa to give you a much-needed protein and health boost. The weight loss potential is awesome, too.

BLACK BEAN QUINOA SALAD: RECIPE 1

"Yummy, and pretty easy to make!"

Ingredients

- 1 cup of quinoa
- 2 cups of water
- 2 to 3 oranges, cut into segments
- 1 red bell pepper, diced
- 1 jalapeno, seeded and diced
- 1 cup of canned black beans, drained and rinsed
- 1/2 a cup of canned corn kernels, drained
- 1/3 of a cup of chopped red onion
- 2 tablespoons of chopped cilantro leaves

For the Orange Vinaigrette:

- 1/4 of a cup of olive oil
- 1/4 of a cup of apple cider vinegar
- 1/4 of a cup of freshly squeezed orange juice
- zest of 1 orange
- 1 tablespoon of honey

Instructions

- In 2 cups of water, cook quinoa in a large saucepan.
- To make the vinaigrette: whisk together the olive oil, the apple cider vinegar, the orange juice, the orange zest and the honey. Now set aside.
- Now combine the quinoa, the oranges, the bell pepper, the jalapeno, the black beans, the corn, the onion, and the cilantro.
- Drizzle vinaigrette on top of the salad and gently toss to combine.

FRESH QUINOA SALAD (ASIAN STYLE): RECIPE 2

"With that Asian inspiration, it's great for entertaining!"

Ingredients

- 1/2 a cup of quinoa
- 1/4 cup of red cabbage (shredded)
- 1/4 cup of red bell pepper (toughly diced)
- 1/4 cup of carrots (grated)
- 1/4 of a cup corn kernels
- 1 green medium sized onion, thinly sliced
- 1 medium avocado, peeled, seeded and diced
- 1/4 of cup noodles Chow Mein variety

For the Sesame Vinaigrette

- 6 tablespoons of rice wine vinegar
- 1 clove of garlic, minced or pressed
- 1 tablespoon of sesame oil
- 1 tablespoon of honey
- 1 teaspoon of low sodium soy sauce
- 1 teaspoon of grated ginger

Instructions

- For the vinaigrette: in a small bowl add together rice wine vinegar, sesame oil, garlic, ginger, honey, and the low-sodium soy sauce. Whisk well and set aside.
- In a medium sized saucepan, cook the quinoa.
- In a large bowl, combine the quinoa, bell pepper, cabbage, carrots, corn kernels, sliced onion, and the avocado.
- Pour in sesame vinaigrette and coat all vegetables well.
- Top with the Chow Mein noodles.

SCRUMPTIOUS QUINOA MEATBALLS: RECIPE 3

"Perfect on cool nights, and so easy to do!"

Ingredients

- 1 lb. of ground turkey breast
- 3/4 of a cup of cooked quinoa
- 3 cloves of garlic, diced finely or minced
- 2 medium green onions, sliced thinly
- 1 egg
- 1 tablespoon of low-sodium soy sauce
- 2 teaspoons of sesame oil
- salt and black pepper, to taste
- 1/2 a teaspoon of sesame seeds

For the Sauce

- ¼ a cup of low-sodium soy sauce
- 2 tablespoons of rice wine vinegar
- 1 tablespoon of freshly grated ginger
- 1 tablespoon of honey
- 1 teaspoon of sesame oil
- 2 teaspoons of cornstarch

Instructions

- Preheat oven to 380 degrees F. Oil a large baking dish (you can coat with nonstick spray).
- In a large bowl, add ground turkey, cooked quinoa, minced garlic, onion, egg, low-sodium soy sauce, and the sesame oil.
- Add salt and pepper, to taste.
- Combine well with clean hands or a wooden mixing spoon.
- Form the mixture into 1 1/4 to 1 1/2-inch balls, it makes around 18-20 meatballs.
- Place meatballs onto your prepared baking dish then bake for 18-20 minutes, or until all the sides have browned and the meat is cooked all the way through.
- For the sauce: in a small saucepan, add together 1/2 a cup of water, low-sodium soy sauce, rice wine vinegar, minced ginger, honey, sesame oil, and stir until it's well mixed.
- In a small bowl, add cornstarch and 1 tablespoon of water. Add

to the low-sodium soy sauce mixture and stir until thickened. This should take around 2 minutes.
• Garnish with the sesame seeds and green onion.

QUINOA AND BROCCOLI CASSEROLE: RECIPE 4

Packed full of goodness, with a terrific flavor too!

Ingredients

• 1 cup of uncooked quinoa
• 1 head of broccoli florets, finely chopped
• 2 tablespoons of virgin olive oil, divided into 2 parts
• 1/3 of a cup of breadcrumbs
• 3 chicken breasts, bones and skin removed, thinly-sliced
• salt and ground black pepper, to taste
• 2 tablespoons of butter, unsalted
• 2 tablespoons of all-purpose flour
• 2 cups of low-fat milk
• 1 and a 1/2 cups of low-fat cheddar cheese, grated and divided
• 1/3 of a cup of natural Greek yogurt

Instructions

• Preheat oven to 350 degrees F. Oil a large baking dish (you can coat with nonstick spray).
• In a large saucepan, add 2 cups of water and cook the quinoa as per the package instructions. In the last 5 minutes of cooking time, add chopped broccoli onto the top and steam until tender and cooked through.
• In a large pan, season your sliced chicken breasts with salt and pepper, adjust according to your taste.
• Place in skillet and cook, turn once, cook until cooked through, around 3-4 minutes each side. Cool before cutting into bite-sized pieces. Set aside.

- Melt butter in the skillet over a medium heat. Add flour and whisk until lightly browned, about 1 minute. Gradually add milk and whisk continually, then cook until slightly thickened, around 3-4 minutes.
- Add the quinoa, broccoli, chicken pieces, 1 cup of low-fat cheddar cheese, and the natural Greek yogurt. Season with salt and pepper, to your taste.
- Spread the broccoli mixture into the oiled baking dish and sprinkle on top (the remaining) 1/2 a cup of cheddar cheese.
- Place in the oven and bake until cheese melts, about 5 to 6 minutes.

Chapter Eleven

THE IMPORTANCE OF ADDING SUPERFOODS AND HERBS

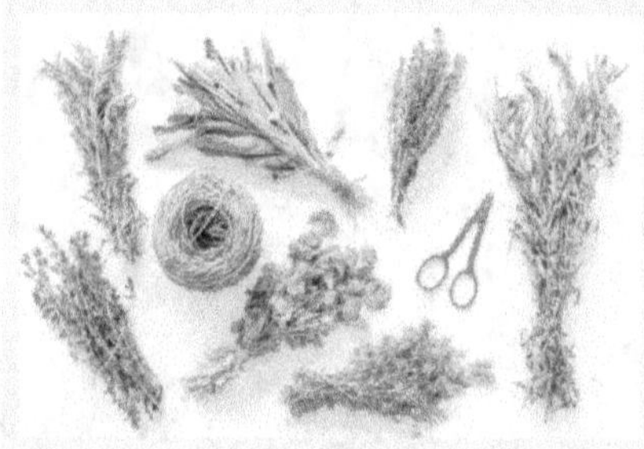

You might have heard the term "superfoods" a few times and wondered what they are, and how they can help you to reach your goal of losing weight.

Why?

All fruits and vegetables come with vitamins, nutrients, and antioxidants, yet superfoods come with a higher number of all of them. They are jam-packed!

A Few Great Examples of Superfoods/Herbs Are:

Gynostemma

This plant originated in Vietnam, Korea, Japan - and most of all China. It became popular in the 1970s. The locals used it as an immortality tea, and when discovered by the western world it was looked at as a substitute for sugar.

When you take this superfood, it is said to harmonize your body and help the individual to regain an inner balance, similar to the way ginseng works.

While studies were being conducted, scientists discovered that it had a concentration of four times the number of saponins when compared to ginseng - and they are called, "gypenosides."

The most common way to take this superfood is by making tea, and it is this tea that helps the metabolic system function better, and it is helpful in removing harmful blood fats, too.

Cinnamon

Cinnamon has been around and used as a spice and flavoring for thousands of years. During this time, it also found its way into being used as a medicine. Not only does cinnamon contain many antioxidants, but it also ranks as one of the highest superfoods to help with blood sugar levels. And it has the benefit of increasing insulin levels and increasing the metabolism of glucose; which is fantastic when you are aiming to lose weight.

These sugars are metabolized before they are "allowed" to turn to fat. The inclusion of cinnamon helps to give that satiated feeling for much longer.

Goji Berries

These little berries are one of the more common superfoods you might have heard of; and for good reason. They have a powerhouse of nutrients and health benefits.

Goji berries are also packed full of polysaccharides, vitamins, minerals, amino acids, and antioxidants to name a few - without containing high levels of fat, or calories. When ingested, the polysaccharides provide probiotic fiber which helps your body to digest food more efficiently and make better use of the nutrients found in other foods.

He Shou Wu

With a rich history in Chinese medicine, he shou wu is in the top sixty superior tonic herbs out of ten thousand, and this herb is regarded as the best longevity provider of them all. One of the most significant contributions it brings to weight loss, is that it helps reduce hepatic fat in the liver. It also helps to fortify muscles while raising overall vitality.

Ginseng Root

Ginseng has to be the most well-known superfood of them all. It has been used for thousands of years in China and other Asian countries. Panax ginseng is the type that is most recommended to include as part of your weight loss regime, because it becomes an adaptogen when ingested.

Ginseng helps to raise the body's metabolism to prevent further buildup of fat, while still reducing glucose and blood sugar levels. When taking ginseng, you might also feel fuller and have much more energy as well.

Gotu Kola

This superfood is not one of the most well-known ones, yet it brings many benefits with it. The most significant advantage is scientists have found it has been found to help with cellulite (mentioned in chapter 9).

Apart from this, gotu kola helps protect the gastrointestinal system and boosts circulation, while having a mild diuretic effect which helps flush wastes from the body.

Acai Berries

These berries sit alongside goji berries as being one of the world's top "superfoods." They were only discovered in the 1990s; deep in the Amazon jungle, where they were a favorite food to the local tribes.

These are another superfood that aid in weight loss by preventing fat buildup within the body. They can also help to boost energy levels, and bring many antiaging benefits with healthy skin being one of them.

Cocoa

There are many health benefits associated with cocoa, and it has been found to contain elements that can help obesity and help individuals to lose weight. This is because it helps to reduce the formation of fatty acids. Although cocoa is high in fat and calories, a small portion is enough for you to gain these benefits from what must be the tastiest superfood, ever. Pure cacao or cacao nibs are full of fiber that aid in the digestive system's functionality.

Wheat Germ

Being one of the world's oldest and most-harvestable crops, wheat germ has stood the test of time as being a superfood, yet the full benefits were not realized until recently, and the healthiest part was often discarded during milling.

Now, wheat germ has been found to provide minerals, vitamins, lots of fiber, omega-3, and complex carbs for the slow release of much-needed energy. To help in your weight loss plan, you can add in wheat germ products as a substitute for processed or refined wheat products.

Pine Pollen

Nature has a funny way of providing us with foods that are healthy and beneficial, and this one is no exception. Actually, this one has been right under our noses, for many years, quite literally so.

Pine pollen is an adaptogen, so it will cater where your body needs it most. It also has a plethora of vitamins which include: vitamin A, most B vitamins, vitamin D, and vitamin E. This is not to mention all the nutrients it contains. One of the main advantages is that it gives a vast amount of protein benefits and includes over twenty, essential, amino acids.

These amazing superfoods and herbs are only the tip of the benefits they bring, yet they offer so much more for weight loss and overall integration for body functioning.

You can also see how easy it is to include them into a juicing practice or in a green smoothie. When combined, or having them as part of a regular meal replacement, you are consuming nothing but pure goodness.

You might have tried to lose weight before and not succeeded as much as you had hoped, yet **when you combine green smoothies with superfoods/herbs and follow a keto way of eating (along with water weight mindfulness)**, your body is defenseless. **It literally can't hang onto those fat deposits that you wish to shift**. That's great news!

As with other foods, you should vary the types of superfoods you choose. Essentially, this broadens the range of benefits you will receive, and once your week-long attempt at losing ten pounds is done, you might find that you crave these superfoods. You should naturally opt for a healthier way of living, long-term. Before you know it, you will have slipped into the keto diet way of living - without any major effort. How good is that?

Chapter Twelve

WEEK PROGRAM

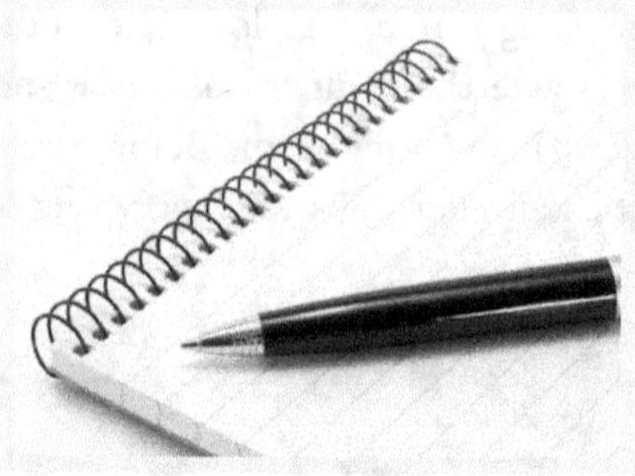

Now, that we've covered everything, I've set out a 7-day plan that you can utilize for yourself. Everything is flexible, and you might need to cater it to your needs due to work or family commitments, too. So, do that and see how great you feel. I am sure it will kick-start your weight loss as it did for me.

Keep in mind, the more often you can utilize a sauna or a steam room, the better, even for only 10 to 15 minutes at a time. Make sure you deep massage any cellulite areas, 5 to 8 minutes is fine, per time. We want to help the body thrive, not stress it. Because stress means that weight placement will go to the abdomen. The body needs to relax as much as it can for weight loss to be achievable. So, adding this activity in as much as you can (3 to 4 times a week, or more) is advisable.

Bike riding can also be fit in anywhere, in the morning, or the afternoon, or evening. As long as it's done once a day for the allocated timeframe of 15 to 20 minutes. This exercise is great for the entire body!

Day 1

Morning:

Nutritional Breakfast - green smoothie or homemade juice, 2 cups of liquid (add 2 eggs if you want)

Activity - stomach rubbing

Activity - bike riding, 20 minutes

Lunchtime:

Nutritional Lunch - quinoa salad and chicken, 1 cup of herbal tea (e.g. chrysanthemum/peppermint)

Activity - stomach rubbing

Dinner:

Nutritional Dinner - beef casserole and green smoothie or homemade juice, 2 cups of liquid

Day 2

Morning:

Nutritional Breakfast - green smoothie or homemade juice, 2 cups of liquid (add eggs and bacon if you want)

Activity - stomach rubbing

Activity - bike riding, 20 minutes

Lunchtime:

Nutritional Lunch - green salad with grilled fish, 1 cup of coffee or herbal tea

Activity - stomach rubbing

Dinner:

Nutritional Dinner - stir-fry chicken with vegetables and a green smoothie or homemade juice, 2 cups of liquid

Day 3

Morning:

Nutritional Breakfast - green smoothie or homemade juice, 2 cups of liquid (add slice of quiche w/quinoa if you want)

Activity - stomach rubbing

Activity - bike riding, 20 minutes

Lunchtime:

Nutritional Lunch - beef and vegetable soup w/salad, and 1 apple/orange, 1 cup of herbal tea (e.g. green tea)

Activity - stomach rubbing

Dinner:

Nutritional Dinner - fish with salad, and green smoothie or homemade juice, 2 cups of liquid

Day 4

Morning:

Nutritional Breakfast - green smoothie or homemade juice, 2 cups of liquid (add 2 eggs if you want)

Activity - stomach rubbing

Activity - bike riding, 20 minutes

Lunchtime:

Nutritional Lunch - garden salad and beef/chicken, 1 cup of coffee or herbal tea (e.g. chrysanthemum)

Activity - stomach rubbing

Dinner:

Nutritional Dinner - steak and green vegetables and green smoothie or homemade juice, 2 cups of liquid

Day 5

Morning:

Nutritional Breakfast - green smoothie or homemade juice, 2 cups of liquid (add 2 eggs if you want)

Activity - stomach rubbing

Activity - bike riding, 20 minutes

Lunchtime:

Nutritional Lunch - chicken stir fry, 1 cup of herbal tea (e.g. chrysanthemum)

Activity - stomach rubbing

Dinner:

Nutritional Dinner - Thai green curry (beef or chicken) and green smoothie or homemade juice, 2 cups of liquid

Day 6

Morning:

Nutritional Breakfast - green smoothie or homemade juice, 2 cups of liquid (add eggs and bacon if you want)

Activity - stomach rubbing

Activity - bike riding, 20 minutes

Lunchtime:

Nutritional Lunch - quinoa salad and chicken, 1 cup tea or coffee

Activity - stomach rubbing

Dinner:

Nutritional Dinner - shrimp and salad and green smoothie or home-made juice, 2 cups of liquid

Day 7

Morning:

Nutritional Breakfast - green smoothie or homemade juice, 2 cups of liquid (add 2 eggs if you want)

Activity - stomach rubbing

Activity - bike riding, 20 minutes

Lunchtime:

Nutritional Lunch - quinoa quiche, 1 cup of herbal tea (e.g. chrysanthemum)

Activity - stomach rubbing

Dinner:

Nutritional Dinner – chicken or beef casserole and green smoothie or homemade juice, 2 cups of liquid

IN CONCLUSION

Thank you for joining me here! I know you can do this... because I did. When you have read through all the chapters, you will see each area is separate, and once you have read it all, you then have to piece together your own, individual plan. This task of losing ten pounds in one week is not easy, yet nothing worth doing, ever is.

By pulling together the very best ways of **cutting out the junk**, and helping your body to perform at its best, you can lose weight without just cutting out food and exercising.

With the inclusion of following the **keto diet eating style**, your body will fall into a state of ketosis - and you will be burning fat while resting. Losing ten pounds would not be possible if it was not for this state the body falls into. **The 6 cups per day rule is also a much-needed practice.** Add in **juicing and green smoothies**, then **the exercise needed to burn the stated calories**.

Hard work always pays off if you do things correctly. **Plan your week and stick to what you have planned, and you will get results**. Each area works together with the other, yet they are all geared to you losing weight and leading a much healthier lifestyle on the whole.

Once you have completed the week, you might find that you have achieved better results than you could have wished for. **It is vital that you come up with a plan first**, for the short period in which you've set to achieve your goal. On a regular diet, you could make it up as you go along, but, a week is not much time to make anything up – so plan ahead of time for success.

Plan it well and before you know it the week will be over... and you will be lighter!

As usual, I am sending you all the luck in the whole, wide world, and I'm always here, cheering you on!

Loads of love, always, *Emma* xx

P.S. You got this!!

Remember!! Some of my best secrets can be found in my title, "How I Lost 100 Pounds! My Personal Weight Loss Strategies for Optimum Happiness." You can see exactly what I did over a 22-month period to lose the weight for good... and keep it off. I now feel better and happier than I've ever felt before. You will learn about the purposeful nutrition you need, balance as a way of eating, a great ancient technique to skyrocket your weight loss, how to lose belly fat, superfoods and herbs, and all about water weight and cellulite removal and prevention. It's totally FREE! Don't forget to get your copy today.

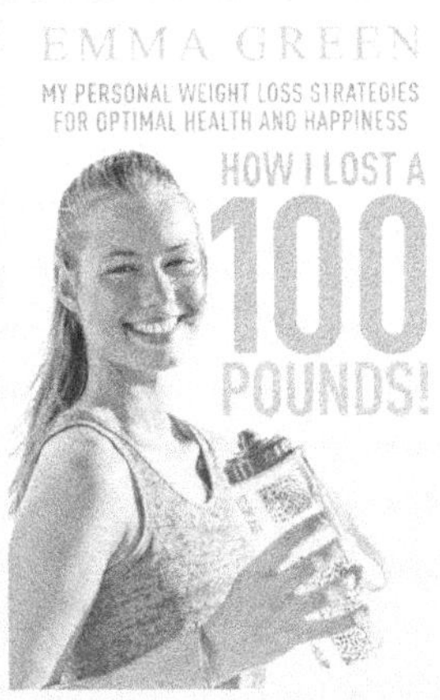

Click here to get your FREE copy! or check out my author profile for other Free titles.